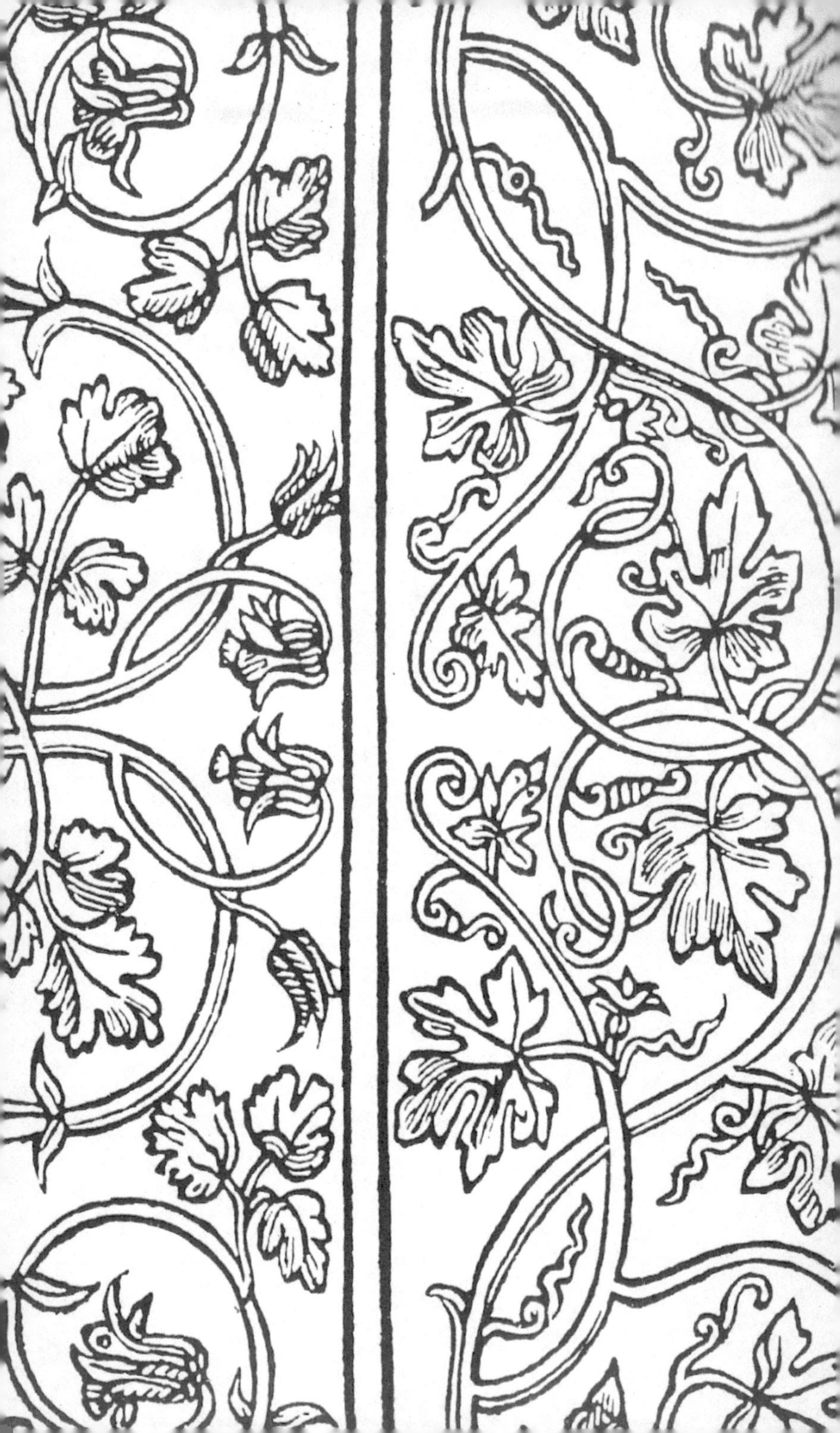

תפלת הרופאים

The Physician's Prayer

Sepher Margaliyyot Tobot

Precious Pearls

Venice 1665

Rabbi Physician

Jacob Ben Isaac Zahalon

of Rome

Reissued by Dr. Aaron J. Feingold

Rosh Hashanah 2022

5783

ISBN # 979-8-3496-6643-8

Published by Bashevis Press in 2025

Zahalon in 1665 urges the physician to recite this prayer at least once a week. It was written after fighting the plague in Rome and describes the physician as acting as agent for the Divine purpose in betterment of Humankind and guided by the most high ethical standards. It is as relevant today as it was in 1665 and always.

Aaron J. Feingold, M.D.

Lord of the Universe! Thou alone has made the Heavens and the Heavens of Heavens and all their hosts, the earth and all that is upon it, the seas and all that is within them. Thou givest life to all and sustenance to all. The hosts of Heavens bow to Thee and there is neither among those on high nor among those underneath anyone who would tell Thee what to do. Thou has formed man from the dust of the ground. Thou has breathed the spirit of life within his nostrils. Thou hast caused him to rule over the works of Thy hand. Everything Thou has placed under his feet. For his sake Thou has created all. If he meritoriously performs the will of his Master, his hand ruleth over all things; if not, the hand of all is upon him.

Thou cost punish him with afflictions and ailments. He is chastened also with pain on his bed and all his bones grow stiff. His flesh is consumed away that it cannot be seen and his bones corrode to unsightliness. His soul draweth near unto the pit and his life to the destroyers. (Job 19, 21, 22, 33). But if he repents completely before Thee, Thou art pleased with him and Thou wilt cure him as it is written: “He sent His word and healed them and delivered them from their graves.”

(Ps. 107:20). For Thou art the merciful and faithful healer, as it is written: “I have wounded and I heal” (Deut. 32:39), in order to make known to all the denizens of the world that Thou art the healer and unto Thee is the power and the glory. From Thy established habitation Thou lookest down upon all the inhabitants of the earth. For their special benefit, has Thou created in Thy world many drugs by which to cure the sons of man and in Thy wisdom Thou has commanded them to cure one another by means of these medicines, as it is written: “He shall cause him to be thoroughly healed.” (Ex. 21:19).

Since, therefore, Thou hast favored me with kindness and has crowned me with honor and glory and Thou hast made me worthy of knowing a bit of the science of medicine, therefore I wish to perform Thy desire, O Lord… I am reminded to busy myself with the practice of medicine in Thy Holy Name and through Thy assistance: “that Thou mayest be justified when Thou speakest and be in the right when Thou judgest" (Ps. 51:6), for Thou art the physician, not I. I am but as the clay in the potter's hand, in the hand of the creator of all things and as the instrument through which Thou curest Thy creatures. I do not rely upon my wisdom, nor do I place my trust in the drugs and herbs and medicaments which Thou has created, for they are but the means to fulfill Thy will and to proclaim Thy greatness and Thy providence. Since the practice of medicine is fraught with perils, and as I am a man of folly and of no understanding fearing lest I grope at noonday as the blind grope in the dark, therefore do I cling to the fringes of Thy kindness and do follow Thee: in the light of Thy countenance will I walk and in Thy light will I behold light. "For Thou cost light my lamp: Lord my God cloth lighten my darkness." (Ps. 18:29). Therefore, may it be Thy will, O Lord my God and God of my fathers to endow me with good understanding... and to bestow upon me knowledge and insight and to cause the eyes of my understanding to shine so that I may discern and diagnose the ailment of the body thoroughly and correctly in all cases that come to me; instruct me as to the drugs suitable to each one in accordance with his needs and in accordance with proper time when they are fit so that I may not err in my acts or in my words, "lest my enemies see and rejoice." (Prov. 24: 17). Support me that I do not stumble and that no mishap occurs through my hands. Recompense me by many kindnesses, for to do kindness have I entered into the profession of medicine, to save lives of Thy people Israel. Assist me and protect me from insult and shame... If there comes to me any patient whose allotted time is about to end and whose affliction is heavy may it be Thy will that I cause not the hastening of his death (God forbid) even by one second. Teach me to administer drugs so as to retain his soul with him until his fated hour arrives. And if he dies may it be Thy will that his friends, his companions and the members of his family do not accuse me and they do not suspect me of being the cause of his death, but that they accept it as a just decree of God of the King in Whose hand is the life of all living and the spirit of all flesh. But if his appointed time has not arrived and Thou art casting him down with pain because of Thy mercy and order that he repent completely before Thee for thou hast “no pleasure in the death of the wicked, but that the wicked turn away from his way and Live” (Ex. 33: 11), may it then be Thy will that Thou causest this merit to fall to my lot and that Thou instructest me what I shall say in order to bring him to repentance and to accept his affliction with love for Thee so that it may be in atonement for all his transgressions; and that through me Thou sendest forth Thy command and cure and that thereby I shalt be beloved on high, and honored below.

Save me from hate and strife. Let me not be envious of others, and may others not envy me. Establish between me and other physicians love, brotherhood, peace and good fellowship. Let me not be put to shame nor disgraced before them, but let me be respected by them. Make me wiser than my enemies. May my wisdom and the knowledge which my lips utter be clear so that there are none to utter an evil word against me or my deeds, and if perchance such evil word be spoken, let no one give it credence. Let not my colleagues err and permit me to rejoice. If, however, they do evil in their work, may it be Thy will to place a muzzle to my mouth and let me not reveal their wrongdoing, but may I have the merit to repair what they have injured. Let me find grace and favor and kindness in Thy eyes and the eyes of all who see me and hear me so that they do what I order for a patient if a treatment is proper, but if the treatment is not proper then harden their hearts that they do not do it, but let them not make it widely known lest (God forbid) I be disgraced O Lord, God of the spirit of all flesh.

I ask one favor of Thee, that Thou give strength to my memory so that when I go to visit a patient, Thou make known to me at once which cures will benefit him whether I have studied it or not. I supplicate Thee, cause of all causes, that Thou cause the chain of circumstances to act in such a manner that Thou bringest into my hands the medical book in which I may study his treatment or that I may listen to an argument between physicians that will teach me to know his cure, for

Thou art the one who brings about the succession of causes in Thy Universe, as it is written: "And they are turned around about his guidance, that they may do whatsoever He commandeth them upon the face of the habitable world." (Job 37:12). I pray Thee O Lord, that Thou bring upon me merit in this world and not demerit. (May God forbid!) Do not cause that any evil thing be found in my hand. Let no corruption come from me, so that I should cause any man's death nor even the loss of his limbs, neither willingly with intent nor unwillingly without interest; let me not be included in the category of the "best physicians are fit for Gehenna" (Mishna Kiddushim IV: 14). "Gather not my soul with sinners, nor my life with men of blood." (Ps. 26:9).

But for the merit which Thou mayest bring to me in that I may preserve lives of Israel, Thy people, whom Thou wilt save from death through me, grant that I may deserve to walk about this world in the pleasure of beholding the good Thy chosen ones, rejoicing in the joy of Thy people, of glorying in Thy inheritance. May my eyes see

Jerusalem, the peaceful habitation. May I walk before the Lord in the land of the living. Let not Satan attach himself to the work of my hand, for to purify and to cleanse I have come! My God, deliver me from the hand of the wicked, from the palm of the pervertor and oppressor and place me not in his hand even for one moment lest he entice me to practice wantonness (God forbid) to administer a poison or drug to injure some man or some pregnant woman (God forbid). If he try to entice me, meet him, humiliate him, deliver my soul from him. "O Lord, I am oppressed, be Thou my surety" (Isaiah 38:14) for Thou art my hope. O Lord God, my trust since my youth. Cleanse my mind and purify my thoughts that I think no evil about any women, whether virgin or wife, when I visit her that do not go about my own heart and my own eyes" (Num. 15:39). Save me from all injury, disease and infirmity... "May the sun not smite me by day nor the moon by night" (Ps. 121:6).

I pray, O Thou Master of kindness and mercy, open my eyes that I may discover the secrets of

Thy wonderful deeds and that I may know the peculiar curative powers which Thou has placed in herbs and minerals, in seeds and flowers, in roots and leaves, in wood and fruit, in wines and oils, in waters and in other liquids, in living organisms which are in the heavens above and in the waters under the earth, in simple and composite structures, and that through them I shall tell of Thy might to all generations to whom Thy greatness shall come. May it be Thy will to give Thy blessing to all the works of my hand and to recompense which is given me against my will so that I may look upon it as an omen of good and that I may apply it to good and righteous purposes before Thee and to magnify and glorify Thy law. And may my sustenance and that of my children and that of my children's children come from Thy hands and not from the hands of men of flesh and blood, and may it be in abundance so that I be not forced to take anything from the poor and sick but, on the contrary, that I may be able to give unto them what Thou hast bestowed upon me, for from Thee come all things and from Thy hands I return to Thee. Endow me well that I succeed and prosper in all that I do, and especially in the work of healing do Thou magnify Thy kindness so that patients call me to whom cure is possible and who may be cured completely through me. And let those not call me who are incurable and whose illness is fatal because Thou hast decreed that they may not be cured. "Let my soul not come unto their council; unto their assembly let my soul not be united" (Gen. 49:6). If people consult me because of my knowledge let not the foot of pride overtake me, but let my soul be "like a weaned child with his mother." (Ps. 131:2). May no evil desire nor vile eye have power over me. Let me not be brought into temptation or shame. Save me from the reflection of sin, and transgression and iniquity, now and forever, and clothe my soul with glorious raiment, the crown of glory of good morals, as is becoming to one who finds grace in Thy eyes. Lend strength to all my senses so that they may tell the truth in everything which is brought before them, that I may not be mistaken in any one of them, neither in taste, smell, signs, hearing nor touch, let them tell me concerning what is positive that it is positive, what is negative,

negative, what is bitter, bitter, sweet, sweet, so that no injury result to any of my patients because of the weakness of my perceptions. Strengthen likewise the power of speech of the patient and the vigor of his understanding and his memory so that he may tell me the truth as to the causes of his ailment and no falsehood in regard to them lest I, also, be led into error and thus fail to understand the causes of his disease from his words and from the symptoms of his disease; let me be fit and learn to prognosticate correctly to the patient in order that my words and warnings may be verified and my injunctions observed. "Uphold me according to Thy word, that I may live; and put me not to shame in my hope" (Ps. 119: 116). Do not destroy hope from out my heart; do not incline me to do evil; do not hide Thyself from my supplications; be gracious unto me and answer me; harken unto my prayer.

Indeed, Thou harkenest unto my prayer and I must give thanks for everything and sing Hallelujahs and praise Thy. name; for goodness is in store for Thy saints' May I increase in greatness and mayest Thou comfort me. May these words which I have supplicated to the Lord come to pass.

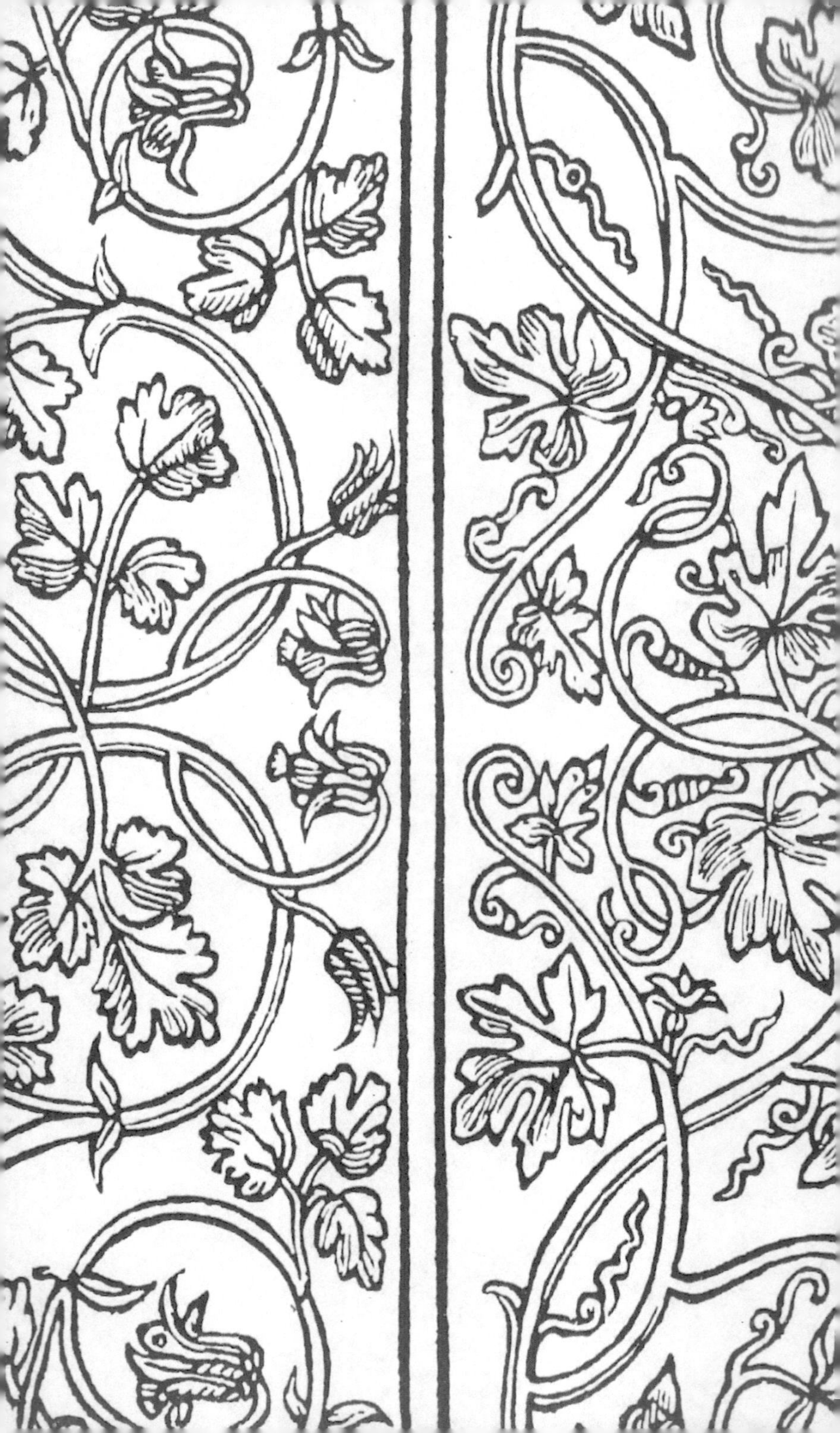

www.ingramcontent.com/pod-product-compliance
Lightning Source LLC
LaVergne TN
LVHW100103250926
848814LV00045B/13